OSTEOPOROSIS DIET COOKBOOK:

1500+ Days of Easy and Simple Low-Carb Delicious Recipes for Men and Women With Osteoporosis

BY

NELSON ROBINSON

TABLE OF CONTENTS

INTRODUCTION..**5**

CHAPTER 1: WELCOME TO THE WORLD OSTEOPOROSIS Cooking...................................... **9**

Understanding Osteoporosis and Nutrition.........9

Importance of a Low-Carb Diet for Bone Health. 15

Basic ingredients in Osteoporosis cooking....... 21

CHAPTER 1: BREAKFAST RECIPES.............**27**

Nutrient-Packed Avocado Omelette.................27

Spinach and Feta Breakfast Casserole............. 29

Chia Seed Pudding with Berries..................... 31

Broccoli and Cheese Egg Muffins................... 33

Smoked Salmon and Cream Cheese Wrap........35

Greek Yogurt Parfait with Almonds and Berries.. 37

CHAPTER 2: LUNCH RECIPES......................**39**

Grilled Chicken Caesar Salad.......................... 39

Quinoa and Vegetable Stuffed Peppers............. 41

Salmon and Asparagus Salad.......................... 43

Turkey and Avocado Lettuce Wraps................. 45

Zucchini Noodles with Pesto and Cherry Tomatoes.. 47

Lentil and Vegetable Soup........................ 49

CHAPTER 3: DINNER RECIPES...................... 51

Baked Cod with Lemon and Herbs................... 51

Cauliflower Crust Margherita Pizza................53

Grilled Tofu and Vegetable Skewers................55

Spaghetti Squash with Meatballs and Marinara 57

Chicken and Broccoli Stir-Fry.......................... 59

Quiche with Spinach and Mushrooms.............. 61

CHAPTER 4: SNACK RECIPES...................... 63

Almond and Cheese Stuffed Jalapeños............. 63

Greek Yogurt Dip with Fresh Veggies.............. 66

Avocado and Tomato Salsa............................. 68

Cucumber and Hummus Bites......................... 70

Roasted Chickpeas with Turmeric and Cumin..72

Cheese and Nut Trail Mix.............................. 74

CONCLUSION....................................... 76

INTRODUCTION

In the intricate tapestry of human health, the significance of a well-balanced and nourishing diet cannot be overstated. As we traverse the realms of nutritional science, there emerges a vital intersection where culinary expertise meets medical understanding—specifically in the context of osteoporosis. Osteoporosis, a condition characterized by weakened and brittle bones, poses a formidable challenge to the skeletal framework that supports our body. It is a silent adversary, often manifesting without noticeable symptoms until fractures occur. In the pursuit of a holistic approach to managing and preventing osteoporosis, the role of thoughtful and purposeful cooking takes center stage.

Beyond merely satisfying our taste buds, cooking becomes a powerful tool in crafting meals that fortify bones, enhance mineral absorption, and foster overall bone health. This intersection of culinary artistry and osteoporosis management delves into a realm where ingredients transform into allies, and recipes evolve into prescriptions. By weaving together the science of nutrition and the art of flavor, we embark on a culinary journey that not only delights the palate but also nourishes the very foundation of our physical well-being.

This exploration delves into the intricacies of osteoporosis cooking, uncovering the nuanced interplay between ingredients, cooking methods, and nutritional value. From calcium-rich culinary creations to vitamin D-infused delights, the palette of osteoporosis-friendly recipes is as diverse as it is delicious. As we navigate this gastronomic expedition, the goal is not just to provide sustenance but to empower individuals with the knowledge to proactively safeguard their bone health.

Join us as we delve into the world of osteoporosis cooking, where every recipe becomes a step towards fortifying our bones, and every meal an investment in a resilient skeletal future. Let the kitchen be your laboratory, and the ingredients your tools, as we embark on a culinary odyssey that transcends the realm of taste, embracing the profound impact that mindful and purposeful cooking can have on the battle against osteoporosis.

CHAPTER 1: WELCOME TO THE WORLD OSTEOPOROSIS Cooking

Understanding Osteoporosis and Nutrition

Welcome to the World Osteoporosis Cooking, where we embark on a journey to explore the intersection of osteoporosis and nutrition. Osteoporosis, a condition characterized by weakened bones, is a global health concern that affects millions of individuals, particularly as they age. While medical interventions play a crucial role in managing and preventing osteoporosis, the significance of nutrition should not be overlooked. This culinary exploration aims to shed light on the role of food in supporting bone health and overall well-being.

Understanding Osteoporosis:

Osteoporosis occurs when the density and quality of bone are reduced, making them fragile and more susceptible to fractures. Bones constantly undergo a process of renewal, where old bone is broken down, and new bone is formed. However, in osteoporosis, the creation of new bone doesn't keep up with the removal of old bone.

Various factors contribute to the development of osteoporosis, including age, genetics, hormonal changes, and lifestyle choices. Women, especially after menopause, are more prone to osteoporosis due to the decline in estrogen levels, which plays a vital role in maintaining bone density.

The Role of Nutrition:

A well-balanced diet rich in essential nutrients is fundamental for maintaining optimal bone health. Key nutrients include:

Calcium: This mineral is a building block for bones. Dairy products, leafy green vegetables, nuts, and fortified foods are excellent sources of calcium.

Vitamin D: Essential for the absorption of calcium, vitamin D is synthesized in the skin when exposed to sunlight. Fatty fish, fortified foods, and supplements are alternative sources.

Protein: Collagen, a protein found in bones, contributes to their strength. Incorporate lean proteins like poultry, fish, beans, and legumes into your meals.

Magnesium: Found in nuts, seeds, whole grains, and green leafy vegetables, magnesium supports bone health by aiding in calcium absorption.

Vitamin K: This vitamin regulates calcium in the bones and blood. Green leafy vegetables, broccoli, and Brussels sprouts are excellent sources.

Osteoporosis-Friendly Recipes:

Salmon and Broccoli Quinoa Bowl:

Rich in omega-3 fatty acids from salmon.

Packed with calcium and vitamin K from broccoli.

Quinoa provides a wholesome source of protein.

Spinach and Feta Stuffed Chicken Breast:

Spinach offers a dose of calcium and vitamin K.

Feta cheese adds a delicious protein boost.

Mango and Kale Smoothie:

Fortified with vitamin D and calcium from fortified plant-based milk.

Kale contributes to the magnesium content.

Greek Yogurt Parfait with Berries:

Greek yogurt is a calcium and protein powerhouse.

Berries add antioxidants and additional vitamins.

Welcome to the World Osteoporosis Cooking, where delicious and nutritious meals become a tool in the fight against osteoporosis. By understanding the impact of nutrition on bone health and incorporating osteoporosis-friendly recipes into our daily lives, we can take proactive steps towards building and maintaining strong, resilient bones. Let's savor the flavors of a bone-healthy lifestyle and nourish our bodies from the inside out.

Importance of a Low-Carb Diet for Bone Health

In the realm of culinary wellness, the World Osteoporosis Cooking initiative invites you to embark on a journey towards stronger bones and overall well-being. Osteoporosis, a condition characterized by the weakening of bones, underscores the importance of adopting a mindful approach to nutrition. One dietary strategy that holds significant promise for bone health is the incorporation of a low-carb diet.

Understanding Osteoporosis: A Call for Nutritional Vigilance

Osteoporosis is a progressive bone disease that leads to increased fragility and susceptibility to fractures. While factors such as age, genetics, and hormonal changes contribute to its onset, lifestyle choices, including diet, play a pivotal role in its prevention and management.

Bones are dynamic structures, constantly undergoing a process of breakdown and rebuilding. Calcium, an essential mineral, serves as a cornerstone in maintaining bone density and strength. The body's ability to absorb calcium, however, can be affected by the presence of certain dietary components, and this is where a low-carb diet comes into play.

The Role of Low-Carb Diets in Bone Health
Low-carbohydrate diets, characterized by reduced intake of sugars and starches, have gained popularity for their impact on various aspects of health. When it comes to bone health, these diets offer several benefits:

Reduced Acid Load: High-carb diets, especially those rich in refined sugars, can lead to increased acidity in the body. This acidic environment prompts the release of calcium from bones to neutralize the pH. Low-carb diets, by contrast, are associated with a lower acid load, preserving calcium in bones.

Stabilized Blood Sugar: Fluctuations in blood sugar levels can negatively affect bone health. Low-carb diets help regulate blood sugar, reducing the risk of insulin spikes that may interfere with optimal bone metabolism.

Weight Management: Maintaining a healthy weight is crucial for bone health. Low-carb diets often facilitate weight loss or weight maintenance, reducing the strain on bones and joints.

Nutrient-Dense Choices: Embracing a low-carb lifestyle encourages the consumption of nutrient-dense foods, such as leafy greens, nuts, seeds, and dairy products. These foods provide essential vitamins and minerals, including calcium and vitamin D, vital for bone health.

Inflammation Reduction: Chronic inflammation is linked to various health issues, including bone loss. Low-carb diets have been associated with a reduction in inflammatory markers, contributing to better overall bone health.

Culinary Adventures for Bone Wellness

Embarking on a low-carb journey doesn't mean sacrificing flavor or variety. Explore the world of osteoporosis-friendly cooking by incorporating:

Leafy Greens: Rich in calcium and other vital nutrients, leafy greens like kale, spinach, and collard greens make excellent additions to low-carb meals.

Lean Proteins: Include sources of lean protein such as poultry, fish, and tofu, providing essential amino acids for bone structure.

Nuts and Seeds: Packed with nutrients, nuts and seeds add a delightful crunch to dishes while contributing to bone health.

Dairy or Dairy Alternatives: Ensure an adequate intake of calcium by incorporating dairy or fortified plant-based alternatives into your low-carb diet.

Colorful Vegetables: A rainbow of vegetables not only adds visual appeal but also provides a diverse array of vitamins and minerals crucial for bone strength.

Nourishing Bones, Nourishing Life

As you embark on the World Osteoporosis Cooking journey, remember that every culinary choice is an opportunity to fortify your bones and enhance your overall well-being. Embracing a low-carb diet, rich in bone-friendly nutrients, empowers you to take an active role in preserving and promoting the health of your skeletal system. Welcome to a world where cooking becomes a celebration of life, health, and resilience against osteoporosis.

Basic ingredients in Osteoporosis cooking

Welcome to the world of Osteoporosis Cooking, where delicious meals are crafted with a focus on promoting bone health and combating the effects of osteoporosis. Osteoporosis is a condition characterized by weakened bones, making them more prone to fractures and breaks. Proper nutrition plays a crucial role in managing and preventing osteoporosis, and that's where Osteoporosis Cooking comes in.

Basic Ingredients in Osteoporosis Cooking:

1. Calcium-Rich Foods:

Include dairy products such as milk, yogurt, and cheese in your diet.

Opt for fortified plant-based milk alternatives like almond or soy milk.

Leafy green vegetables like kale, collard greens, and broccoli are excellent sources of calcium. Canned fish with bones, such as sardines and salmon, provide a significant calcium boost.

2. Vitamin D Sources:

Vitamin D is essential for calcium absorption. Include foods rich in vitamin D, like fatty fish (salmon, mackerel), egg yolks, and fortified foods.
Spend some time in the sun to naturally produce vitamin D in your body.

3. Magnesium-Rich Foods:

Magnesium is crucial for bone health and can be found in nuts, seeds, whole grains, and green leafy vegetables.
Include foods like almonds, cashews, spinach, and quinoa in your meals.

4. Protein-Packed Options:

Protein is essential for bone health, and sources like lean meats, poultry, fish, eggs, and plant-based proteins (beans, lentils, tofu) should be included.

Maintain a balanced diet with adequate protein to support bone density.

5. Vitamin K-Enriched Foods:

Vitamin K aids in bone mineralization and can be found in leafy green vegetables like kale, spinach, and Brussels sprouts.

Include a variety of these vegetables in your salads, stir-fries, or smoothies.

6. Phosphorus Sources:

Phosphorus is another mineral vital for bone health. Include foods like dairy products, fish, poultry, and nuts in your diet.

Whole grains such as brown rice and whole wheat also contribute to phosphorus intake.

7. Limit Sodium and Caffeine:

Excessive sodium can lead to calcium loss from the bones. Keep salt intake in check by using herbs and spices for flavor.

Limit caffeine, as high consumption may interfere with calcium absorption. Opt for herbal teas or decaffeinated options.

8. Hydration:

Water is crucial for overall health, including bone health. Ensure you stay hydrated for optimal bodily functions.

9. Regular Exercise:

While not an ingredient, regular weight-bearing exercises like walking, jogging, or strength training complement a bone-healthy diet.

10. Bone-Building Supplements:

Consult with a healthcare professional to determine if calcium or vitamin D supplements are necessary for your specific needs.

In the world of Osteoporosis Cooking, these basic ingredients form the foundation for creating flavorful and nutritious meals that support bone health. By incorporating these elements into your daily diet, you can take a proactive approach to managing osteoporosis and promoting overall well-being. Remember to consult with a healthcare professional or a nutritionist for personalized advice based on your individual needs and health status.

CHAPTER 1: BREAKFAST RECIPES

Nutrient-Packed Avocado Omelette

Time Frame: 10 minutes

Ingredients:

1. 2 eggs
2. 1/2 avocado, sliced
3. 1/4 cup diced tomatoes
4. 1/4 cup diced bell peppers
5. Salt and pepper to taste
6. 1 tablespoon olive oil

Instructions:

1. *In a bowl, beat the eggs and season with salt and pepper.*
2. *Heat olive oil in a non-stick skillet over medium heat.*
3. *Pour the beaten eggs into the skillet and let them set for a minute.*
4. *Add sliced avocado, diced tomatoes, and bell peppers on one side of the omelette.*
5. *Gently fold the other half over the vegetables.*
6. *Cook for another 2-3 minutes until the omelette is cooked through.*
7. *Serve hot and enjoy!*

Tip:

1. *Add a sprinkle of feta cheese or a dollop of Greek yogurt for extra flavor.*

Spinach and Feta Breakfast Casserole

Time Frame: 40 minutes

Ingredients:

1. *6 eggs*

2. *1 cup spinach, chopped*

3. *1/2 cup feta cheese, crumbled*

4. *1/2 cup milk*

5. *Salt and pepper to taste*

6. *1/2 teaspoon garlic powder*

7. *1 tablespoon olive oil*

Instructions:

1. *Preheat the oven to 375°F (190°C).*

2. *In a skillet, sauté spinach in olive oil until wilted.*

3. *In a bowl, whisk together eggs, milk, salt, pepper, and garlic powder.*

4. *Grease a baking dish and spread the sautéed spinach evenly.*

5. *Pour the egg mixture over the spinach and sprinkle feta cheese on top.*

6. *Bake for 25-30 minutes or until the casserole is set and golden.*

7. *Allow it to cool slightly before slicing and serving.*

Tip:

1. *Serve with a side of fresh fruit for a well-balanced breakfast.*

Chia Seed Pudding with Berries

Time Frame: Overnight (or at least 4 hours)

Ingredients:

1. 1/4 cup chia seeds

2. 1 cup almond milk

3. 1 tablespoon honey or maple syrup

4. 1/2 teaspoon vanilla extract

5. Mixed berries for topping

Instructions:

1. *In a bowl, mix chia seeds, almond milk, honey or maple syrup, and vanilla extract.*

2. *Stir well and refrigerate overnight or for at least 4 hours.*

3. *Before serving, give it a good stir and top with fresh berries.*

Tip:

1. *Add a handful of granola or nuts for added crunch.*

Broccoli and Cheese Egg Muffins

Time Frame: 25 minutes

Ingredients:

6 eggs

1 cup broccoli, finely chopped

1/2 cup shredded cheddar cheese

Salt and pepper to taste

Cooking spray

Instructions:

1. *Preheat the oven to 350°F (175°C).*
2. *In a bowl, whisk together eggs, chopped broccoli, shredded cheese, salt, and pepper.*
3. *Grease a muffin tin with cooking spray.*

4. *Pour the egg mixture evenly into the muffin cups.*

5. *Bake for 15-20 minutes or until the egg muffins are set.*

6. *Allow them to cool slightly before removing from the tin.*

Tip:

1. *Make a batch and store them in the fridge for a quick breakfast throughout the week.*

Smoked Salmon and Cream Cheese Wrap

Time Frame: 10 minutes

Ingredients:

1. *1 whole wheat tortilla*

2. *2 ounces smoked salmon*

3. *2 tablespoons cream cheese*

4. *1 tablespoon capers*

5. *Fresh dill for garnish*

Instructions:

1. *Spread cream cheese evenly over the tortilla.*

2. *Layer smoked salmon on top of the cream cheese.*

3. *Sprinkle capers and fresh dill over the salmon.*

4. *Roll the tortilla into a wrap and slice in half.*

Tip:

1. *Serve with a wedge of lemon for an extra burst of flavor.*

Greek Yogurt Parfait with Almonds and Berries

Time Frame: 5 minutes

Ingredients:

1. *1 cup Greek yogurt*
2. *1/4 cup granola*
3. *1/4 cup sliced almonds*
4. *1/2 cup mixed berries (strawberries, blueberries, raspberries)*

Instructions:

1. *In a glass or bowl, layer Greek yogurt, granola, almonds, and mixed berries.*
2. *Repeat the layers until the container is filled.*
3. *Top with a few extra berries and a sprinkle of almonds.*

Tip:

1. *Drizzle with honey for a touch of sweetness.*

CHAPTER 2: LUNCH RECIPES

Grilled Chicken Caesar Salad

Time Frame: 30 minutes

Ingredients:

1. *2 boneless, skinless chicken breasts*
2. *Romaine lettuce, chopped*
3. *1/2 cup cherry tomatoes, halved*
4. *1/4 cup grated Parmesan cheese*
5. *Caesar dressing*
6. *Croutons*

Instructions:

1. *Season chicken breasts with salt and pepper, then grill until fully cooked.*
2. *Slice the grilled chicken into strips.*

3. *In a large bowl, toss chopped romaine lettuce, cherry tomatoes, and grilled chicken.*

4. *Sprinkle Parmesan cheese over the salad.*

5. *Drizzle Caesar dressing and toss until well-coated.*

6. *Top with croutons before serving.*

Tip:

1. *For an extra kick, sprinkle with freshly ground black pepper and additional Parmesan.*

Quinoa and Vegetable Stuffed Peppers

Time Frame: 45 minutes

Ingredients:

1. *4 bell peppers, halved and seeds removed*
2. *1 cup quinoa, cooked*
3. *1 can black beans, drained and rinsed*
4. *1 cup corn kernels*
5. *1 cup diced tomatoes*
6. *1 cup shredded cheddar cheese*
7. *Taco seasoning*
8. *Fresh cilantro for garnish*

Instructions:

1. *Preheat the oven to 375°F (190°C).*

2. *In a large bowl, mix cooked quinoa, black beans, corn, diced tomatoes, and taco seasoning.*

3. *Stuff each pepper half with the quinoa mixture.*

4. *Top with shredded cheddar cheese.*

5. *Bake for 25-30 minutes or until peppers are tender.*

6. *Garnish with fresh cilantro before serving.*

Tip:

1. *Serve with a dollop of Greek yogurt or salsa on top.*

Salmon and Asparagus Salad

Time Frame: 20 minutes

Ingredients:

1. *2 salmon fillets*
2. *1 bunch asparagus, trimmed*
3. *Mixed greens*
4. *Cherry tomatoes, halved*
5. *Balsamic vinaigrette*
6. *Lemon wedges*

Instructions:

1. *Season salmon fillets with salt and pepper, then grill or pan-sear until cooked.*
2. *In a pot of boiling water, blanch asparagus for 2-3 minutes.*

3. *Assemble mixed greens on a plate, top with cherry tomatoes, grilled salmon, and asparagus.*

4. *Drizzle with balsamic vinaigrette.*

5. *Serve with lemon wedges on the side.*

Tip:

1. *Add a sprinkle of toasted pine nuts for extra crunch.*

Turkey and Avocado Lettuce Wraps

Time Frame: 15 minutes

Ingredients:

1. 1 pound ground turkey
2. 1 tablespoon olive oil
3. Taco seasoning
4. Iceberg lettuce leaves
5. Avocado, sliced
6. Salsa
7. Shredded cheese

Instructions:

1. In a skillet, heat olive oil, add ground turkey, and cook until browned.
2. Season turkey with taco seasoning.

3. *Assemble lettuce wraps with seasoned turkey, avocado slices, salsa, and shredded cheese.*

4. *Serve immediately.*

Tip:

1. *Add a squeeze of lime for a burst of citrus flavor.*

Zucchini Noodles with Pesto and Cherry Tomatoes

Time Frame: 20 minutes

Ingredients:

1. *4 medium zucchinis, spiralized into noodles*
2. *Pesto sauce (store-bought or homemade)*
3. *Cherry tomatoes, halved*
4. *Parmesan cheese, grated*
5. *Pine nuts (optional)*

Instructions:

1. *In a pan, sauté zucchini noodles until just tender.*
2. *Toss the zucchini noodles with pesto sauce.*

3. *Add cherry tomatoes and toss until heated through.*

4. *Top with grated Parmesan cheese and pine nuts if desired.*

5. *Serve warm.*

Tip:

1. *Customize with grilled chicken or shrimp for added protein.*

Lentil and Vegetable Soup

Time Frame: 1 hour

Ingredients:

1. *1 cup dried green or brown lentils, rinsed*
2. *1 onion, diced*
3. *2 carrots, diced*
4. *2 celery stalks, diced*
5. *3 cloves garlic, minced*
6. *1 can diced tomatoes*
7. *6 cups vegetable or chicken broth*
8. *1 teaspoon dried thyme*
9. *Salt and pepper to taste*
10. *Fresh parsley for garnish*

Instructions:

1. *In a large pot, sauté onion, carrots, celery, and garlic until softened.*
2. *Add lentils, diced tomatoes, broth, thyme, salt, and pepper.*
3. *Bring to a boil, then reduce heat and simmer for 30-40 minutes or until lentils are tender.*
4. *Adjust seasoning if needed.*
5. *Garnish with fresh parsley before serving.*

Tip:

1. *Serve with a slice of crusty bread for a complete meal.*

CHAPTER 3: DINNER RECIPES

Baked Cod with Lemon and Herbs

Time Frame: 25 minutes

Ingredients:

1. *4 cod fillets*

2. *2 tablespoons olive oil*

3. *1 lemon, sliced*

4. *2 cloves garlic, minced*

5. *Fresh herbs (such as parsley, thyme, or dill)*

6. *Salt and pepper to taste*

Instructions:

1. *Preheat the oven to 400°F (200°C).*

2. *Place cod fillets on a baking sheet.*

3. *Drizzle olive oil over the fillets and season with salt, pepper, and minced garlic.*

4. *Lay lemon slices on top of the fillets and sprinkle fresh herbs.*

5. *Bake for 15-20 minutes or until the cod flakes easily with a fork.*

6. *Serve hot.*

Tip:

1. *Squeeze extra lemon juice before serving for a burst of citrus flavor.*

Cauliflower Crust Margherita Pizza

Time Frame: 40 minutes

Ingredients:

1. *1 cauliflower head, grated or processed into "rice"*
2. *1 egg*
3. *1 cup mozzarella cheese, shredded*
4. *1 teaspoon dried oregano*
5. *Salt and pepper to taste*
6. *Tomato sauce*
7. *Fresh mozzarella, sliced*
8. *Fresh basil leaves*

Instructions:

1. *Preheat the oven to 425°F (220°C).*

2. *Mix cauliflower rice, egg, mozzarella, oregano, salt, and pepper in a bowl.*

3. *Spread the mixture on a baking sheet, forming a crust.*

4. *Bake for 20 minutes or until the crust is golden.*

5. *Spread tomato sauce over the crust, add fresh mozzarella slices, and sprinkle with fresh basil.*

6. *Bake for an additional 10 minutes or until the cheese is melted.*

Tip:

1. *Ensure the cauliflower crust is well-baked to achieve a crispy texture.*

Grilled Tofu and Vegetable Skewers

Time Frame: 30 minutes (plus marinating time)

Ingredients:

1. *1 block extra-firm tofu, pressed and cubed*
2. *Assorted vegetables (bell peppers, cherry tomatoes, zucchini, mushrooms)*
3. *Marinade: soy sauce, olive oil, garlic, ginger, and a splash of maple syrup*

Instructions:

1. *Mix the marinade ingredients in a bowl.*
2. *Marinate tofu cubes in the mixture for at least 30 minutes.*
3. *Thread tofu cubes and vegetables onto skewers.*

4. *Grill for 15-20 minutes, turning occasionally, until tofu is golden and vegetables are tender.*

5. *Serve hot.*

Tip:

1. *Brush with extra marinade during grilling for added flavor.*

Spaghetti Squash with Meatballs and Marinara

Time Frame: 1 hour

Ingredients:

1. *1 large spaghetti squash, halved and seeds removed*

2. *Meatballs (store-bought or homemade)*

3. *Marinara sauce*

4. *Fresh basil for garnish*

5. *Parmesan cheese, grated*

Instructions:

1. *Preheat the oven to 375°F (190°C).*

2. *Place spaghetti squash halves on a baking sheet, cut side down.*

3. *Bake for 40-45 minutes or until squash is tender.*

4. *While the squash is baking, prepare meatballs and warm marinara sauce.*

5. *Scrape the cooked squash with a fork to create "spaghetti" strands.*

6. *Top with meatballs, marinara sauce, fresh basil, and grated Parmesan.*

Tip:

1. *Roast the spaghetti squash with a drizzle of olive oil for added flavor.*

Chicken and Broccoli Stir-Fry

Time Frame: 20 minutes

Ingredients:

1. *1 lb chicken breast, sliced*
2. *2 cups broccoli florets*
3. *1 red bell pepper, sliced*
4. *2 tablespoons soy sauce*
5. *1 tablespoon oyster sauce*
6. *1 tablespoon sesame oil*
7. *2 cloves garlic, minced*
8. *Ginger, grated*
9. *Rice or noodles for serving*

Instructions:

1. *Heat sesame oil in a wok or skillet over medium-high heat.*

2. *Stir-fry chicken until browned, then add garlic and ginger.*

3. *Add broccoli and bell pepper, stir-fry for a few minutes until vegetables are tender-crisp.*

4. *Mix soy sauce and oyster sauce, then pour over the chicken and vegetables.*

5. *Stir to combine and cook for an additional 2-3 minutes.*

6. *Serve over rice or noodles.*

Tip:

1. *Customize with your favorite stir-fry sauce or add cashews for extra crunch.*

Quiche with Spinach and Mushrooms

Time Frame: 1 hour

Ingredients:

1. *Pie crust (store-bought or homemade)*
2. *1 cup spinach, chopped*
3. *1 cup mushrooms, sliced*
4. *1 cup shredded Swiss cheese*
5. *4 eggs*
6. *1 cup milk*
7. *Salt and pepper to taste*
8. *Nutmeg (optional)*

Instructions:

1. *Preheat the oven to 375°F (190°C).*
2. *In a skillet, sauté spinach and mushrooms until cooked.*

3. *Place the pie crust in a pie dish and spread the sautéed vegetables evenly.*

4. *Sprinkle shredded Swiss cheese over the vegetables.*

5. *In a bowl, whisk together eggs, milk, salt, and pepper.*

6. *Pour the egg mixture over the vegetables and cheese.*

7. *Bake for 35-40 minutes or until the quiche is set and golden.*

8. *Allow it to cool slightly before slicing.*

Tip:

1. *Grate a touch of nutmeg into the egg mixture for a warm, aromatic flavor.*

CHAPTER 4: SNACK RECIPES

Almond and Cheese Stuffed Jalapeños

Time Frame: 25 minutes

Ingredients:

1. *12 fresh jalapeños, halved and seeds removed*
2. *1 cup cream cheese, softened*
3. *1/2 cup shredded cheddar cheese*
4. *1/2 cup almonds, chopped*
5. *1 teaspoon garlic powder*
6. *1 teaspoon onion powder*
7. *Salt and pepper to taste*
8. *Fresh cilantro for garnish (optional)*

Instructions:

1. *Preheat the oven to 375°F (190°C).*

2. *In a bowl, mix cream cheese, shredded cheddar, chopped almonds, garlic powder, onion powder, salt, and pepper until well combined.*

3. *Stuff each jalapeño half with the cheese and almond mixture.*

4. *Place stuffed jalapeños on a baking sheet.*

5. *Bake for 15-20 minutes or until the jalapeños are softened and the filling is golden.*

6. *Garnish with fresh cilantro if desired.*

7. *Allow them to cool slightly before serving.*

Tip:

1. *Wear gloves while handling jalapeños, and adjust the amount of cream cheese for your desired level of heat.*

Greek Yogurt Dip with Fresh Veggies

Time Frame: 10 minutes

Ingredients:

1. *1 cup Greek yogurt*

2. *1 tablespoon olive oil*

3. *1 clove garlic, minced*

4. *1 teaspoon dried dill*

5. *Salt and pepper to taste*

6. *Assorted fresh veggies (carrot sticks, cucumber slices, cherry tomatoes)*

Instructions:

1. *In a bowl, mix Greek yogurt, olive oil, minced garlic, dried dill, salt, and pepper.*

2. *Stir until well combined.*

3. *Chill in the refrigerator for at least 30 minutes.*

4. *Serve the dip with fresh veggies for dipping.*

Tip:

1. *Garnish with additional dill or a drizzle of olive oil before serving.*

Avocado and Tomato Salsa

Time Frame: 15 minutes

Ingredients:

1. *2 ripe avocados, diced*
2. *1 cup cherry tomatoes, halved*
3. *1/4 cup red onion, finely chopped*
4. *1/4 cup fresh cilantro, chopped*
5. *Juice of 1 lime*
6. *Salt and pepper to taste*
7. *Tortilla chips for serving*

Instructions:

1. *In a bowl, combine diced avocados, cherry tomatoes, red onion, and cilantro.*
2. *Squeeze lime juice over the mixture and gently toss.*
3. *Season with salt and pepper to taste.*

4. *Allow the salsa to sit for a few minutes before serving.*

5. *Serve with tortilla chips or as a topping for grilled meats or fish.*

Tip:

1. *Add a pinch of cayenne pepper for a hint of spice.*

Cucumber and Hummus Bites

Time Frame: 15 minutes

Ingredients:

1. English cucumbers, sliced
2. Hummus
3. Cherry tomatoes, halved
4. Kalamata olives, pitted and sliced
5. Fresh parsley, chopped

Instructions:

1. Slice the cucumbers into rounds.
2. Spoon a small amount of hummus onto each cucumber round.
3. Top with a halved cherry tomato and a slice of Kalamata olive.
4. Garnish with fresh parsley.

5. *Arrange on a serving platter and serve chilled.*

Tip:

1. *Drizzle a touch of olive oil over the bites before serving.*

Roasted Chickpeas with Turmeric and Cumin

Time Frame: 40 minutes

Ingredients:

1. *2 cans chickpeas, drained and rinsed*

2. *2 tablespoons olive oil*

3. *1 teaspoon ground turmeric*

4. *1 teaspoon ground cumin*

5. *1/2 teaspoon cayenne pepper*

6. *Salt to taste*

Instructions:

1. *Preheat the oven to 400°F (200°C).*

2. *Pat dry the chickpeas with a paper towel to remove excess moisture.*

3. *In a bowl, toss chickpeas with olive oil, turmeric, cumin, cayenne pepper, and salt.*

4. *Spread the chickpeas in a single layer on a baking sheet.*

5. *Roast for 30-35 minutes or until crispy, shaking the pan occasionally.*

6. *Allow them to cool before serving.*

Tip:

1. *Roasted chickpeas can be a crunchy snack or a salad topper.*

Cheese and Nut Trail Mix

Time Frame: 5 minutes

Ingredients:

1. *1 cup mixed nuts (almonds, walnuts, cashews)*
2. *1 cup cheese cubes (cheddar, mozzarella, or your choice)*
3. *1/2 cup dried fruit (raisins, cranberries, apricots)*

Instructions:

1. *In a bowl, mix together mixed nuts, cheese cubes, and dried fruit.*
2. *Toss until evenly distributed.*
3. *Portion into small snack bags for a quick grab-and-go option.*

Tip:

1. *For added flavor, choose a variety of cheeses like smoked Gouda or pepper jack.*

CONCLUSION

In conclusion, the "Osteoporosis Diet Cookbook: 1500+ Days of Easy and Simple Low-Carb Delicious Recipes for Men and Women with Osteoporosis" serves as a comprehensive and invaluable resource for individuals navigating the challenges of osteoporosis. As we journey through its pages, the cookbook not only offers a diverse array of tantalizing low-carb recipes but also empowers readers with the knowledge and tools necessary to make informed dietary choices that support bone health.

One of the standout features of this cookbook is its commitment to simplicity and ease, recognizing the often overwhelming nature of managing a condition like osteoporosis. The 1500+ recipes included are not only delicious but are designed to be accessible to individuals of varying culinary skill levels. This thoughtful approach ensures that even those with limited experience in the kitchen can embark on a flavorful and osteoporosis-friendly culinary adventure.

The emphasis on low-carb options aligns with contemporary dietary trends while addressing the specific needs of individuals with osteoporosis. The cookbook skillfully navigates the delicate balance of providing nutrient-dense and bone-boosting recipes without sacrificing taste or variety. This not only makes the dietary adjustments more palatable for those with osteoporosis but also encourages a sustainable and enjoyable long-term commitment to bone health.

Beyond the recipes themselves, the book serves as an educational tool, equipping readers with essential information about the role of nutrition in osteoporosis management. It delves into the significance of key nutrients such as calcium, vitamin D, and protein, offering a nuanced understanding of how these elements contribute to bone health. The inclusion of practical tips and guidelines further enhances the educational value of the cookbook, empowering readers to make informed choices beyond the kitchen.

Moreover, the cookbook recognizes the importance of gender-specific considerations in osteoporosis management, catering to the distinct dietary needs of both men and women. This attention to diversity reflects a commitment to inclusivity, acknowledging that osteoporosis affects individuals across a spectrum of age, gender, and lifestyle.

In essence, the "Osteoporosis Diet Cookbook" transcends its role as a mere collection of recipes, emerging as a holistic guide for those navigating the complex terrain of osteoporosis. By combining culinary creativity with nutritional expertise, it transforms the often-daunting task of managing a chronic condition into an opportunity for delicious and healthful exploration. Whether you are someone with osteoporosis, a caregiver, or a healthcare professional seeking practical dietary recommendations, this cookbook stands as an indispensable companion on the journey to better bone health.